Author

Manuel Fernández Sánchez

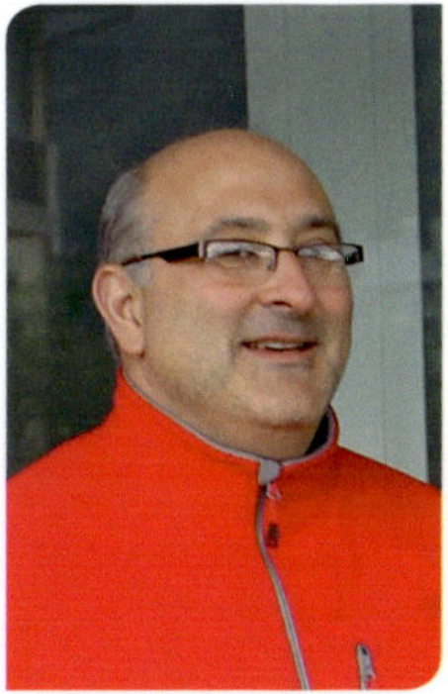

Graduated in veterinary medicine from the University of Zaragoza.

Freelance veterinary consultant. He has worked at ANGRA (the Spanish National Association of Rasa Aragonesa Pedigree Breeders) on the development of programmes for genetic improvement and reproduction in mutton sheep, as well as in Asturias on reproduction monitoring and cow milk quality. He has also participated as a speaker on various courses organised by the University of Santiago de Compostela.

TABLE OF CONTENTS

Reproductive evaluation and ultrasound diagnosis

1 INTRODUCTION 3

2 REPRODUCTIVE PHYSIOLOGY 10

Anatomical knowledge 10
Functional knowledge 12
Hypothalamic-pituitary-gonadal axis 13
Follicular waves 16
Phases of each wave of follicular growth 18

3 ASSESSMENT AND DIAGNOSIS OF REPRODUCTIVE STATUS 24

Methodology 25
Assessment 25
Evaluation 25
Assessment of the uterus 26
Case studies 28

Introduction

- Ultrasound allows better management of key parameters to ensure more effective reproductive control in livestock.
- The starting point is a thorough knowledge of reproductive physiology.
- The result is the diagnosis and evaluation of the uterus and ovaries by ultrasound.

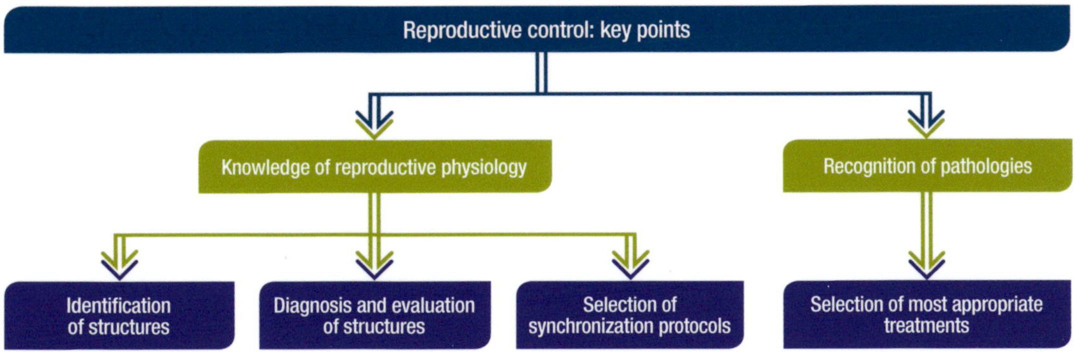

Figure 1. With the development of ultrasound and its increasingly widespread application in cattle, diagnostic and treatment efficiency has increased.

Identification of ovarian structures: corpora lutea

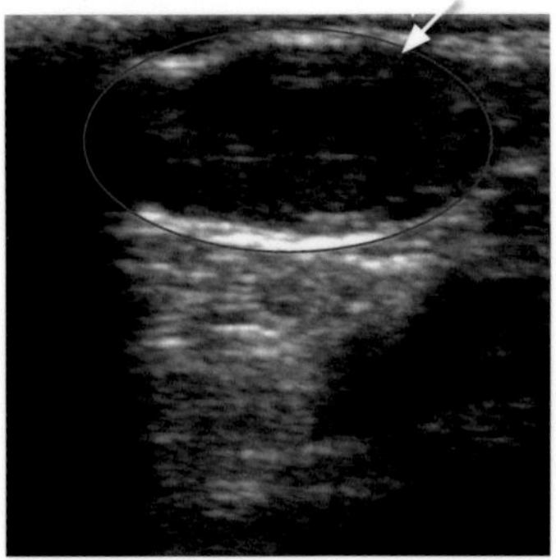

Figure 2. Corpus luteum with trabecula (red line).

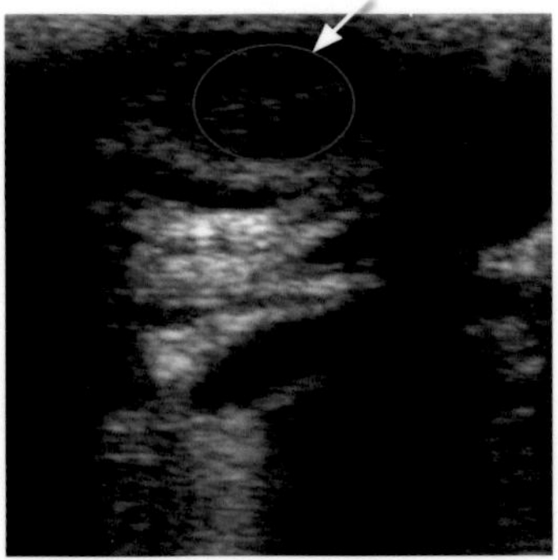

Figure 3. Young corpus luteum (recently ovulated female): sonographically less echogenic than previous image.

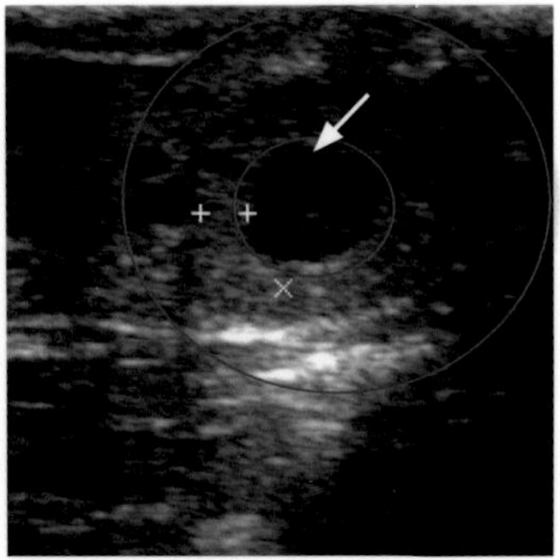

Figure 4. Corpus luteum cyst (with cavity): physiologic.

Choosing synchronisation protocols (e.g. ovsynch)

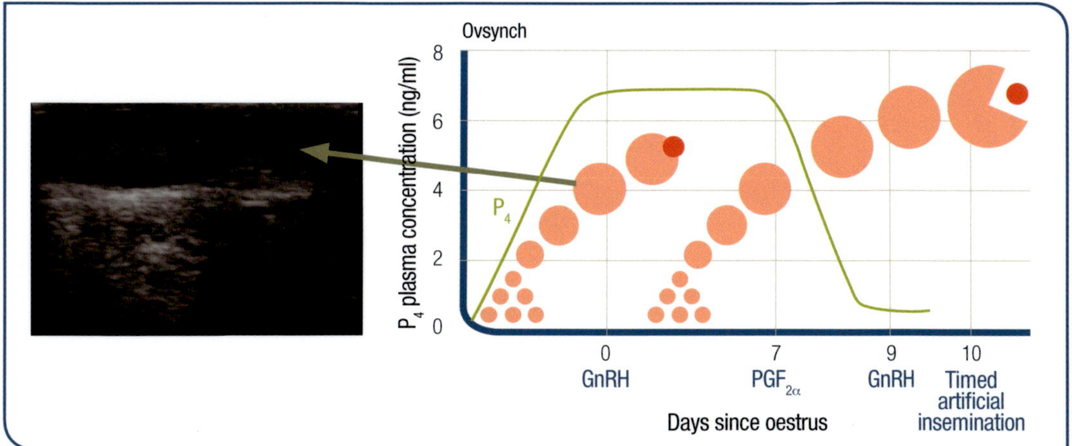

Figure 5. Correct synchronisation of ovsynch treatment: day 6 of cycle = day 0 of treatment (selection phase: first follicular wave).

Recognising pathologies

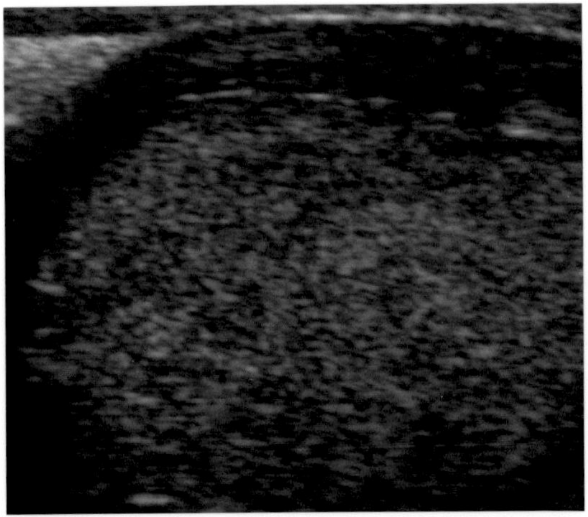

Figure 6. Uterus with abundant purulent material (cloud of dots) in a case of metritis.

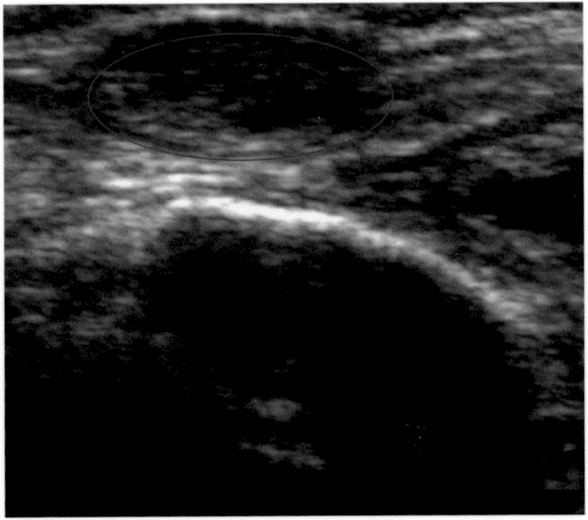

Figure 7. Ovary in anoestrus (no structures).

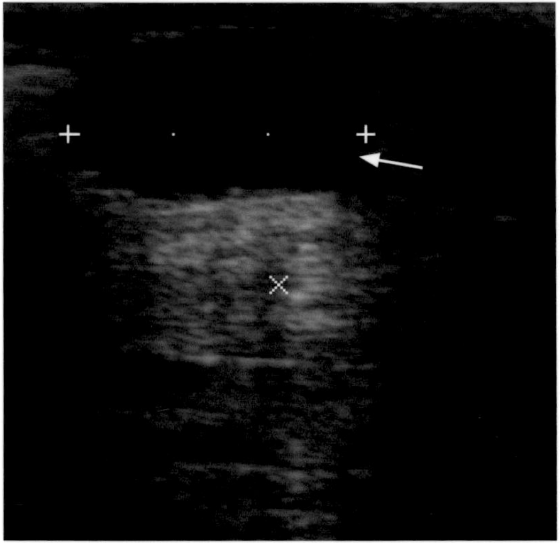

Figure 8. Measurement of follicular cyst (3.1 cm).

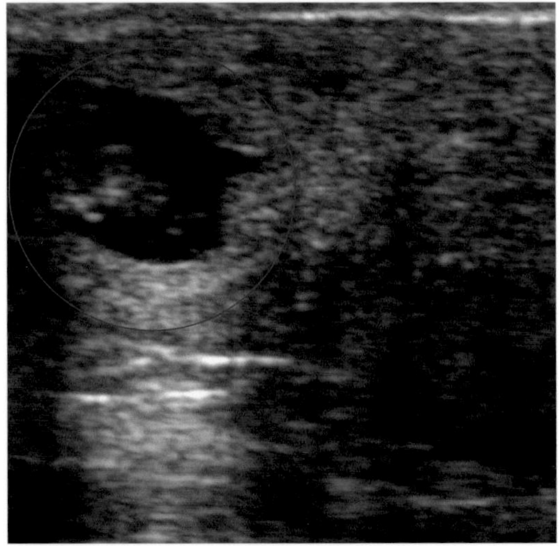

Figure 9. Embryonic resorption (disorganised content).

Selection and evaluation of treatments

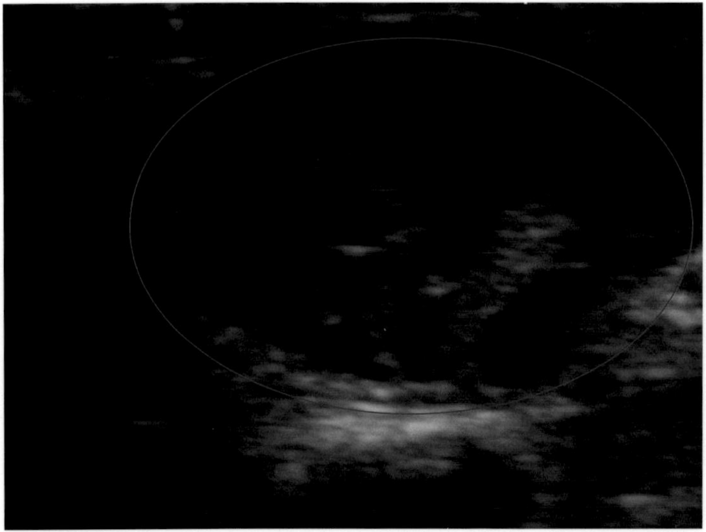

Figure 10. Follicular cyst after 7 days of treatment with GnRH (luteinisation of cyst).

Anatomical knowledge

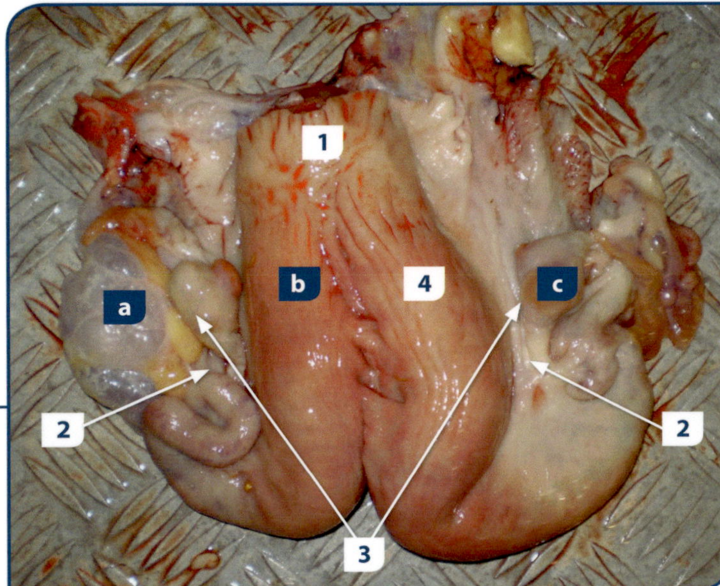

1. Body of uterus.
2. Oviduct.
3. Ovaries.
4. Uterine horns.

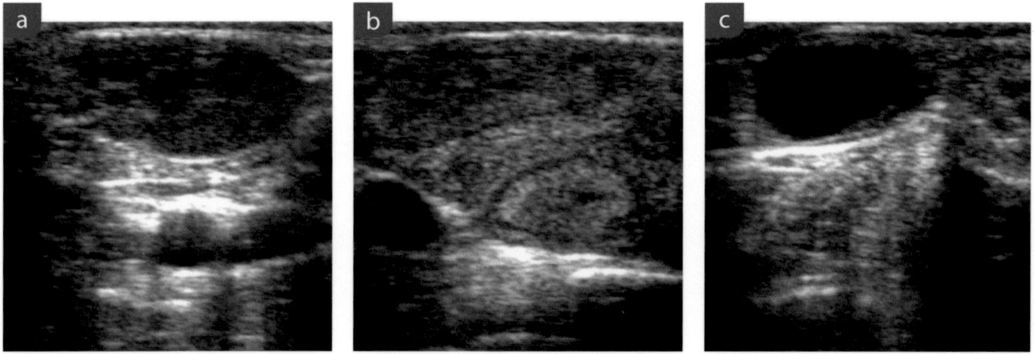

Figure 11. Ultrasound of (a) the corpus luteum, (b) uterine horns and (c) follicle.

Functional knowledge

- It is essential to have a proper understanding of the endocrinological basis of different situations in order to select the best oestrus synchronisation system or the most appropriate treatment for a particular disease.
- The cascade of hormonal events resulting from the intimate relationship between the nervous and endocrine systems is conditioned by multiple stimuli from the environment surrounding the female.

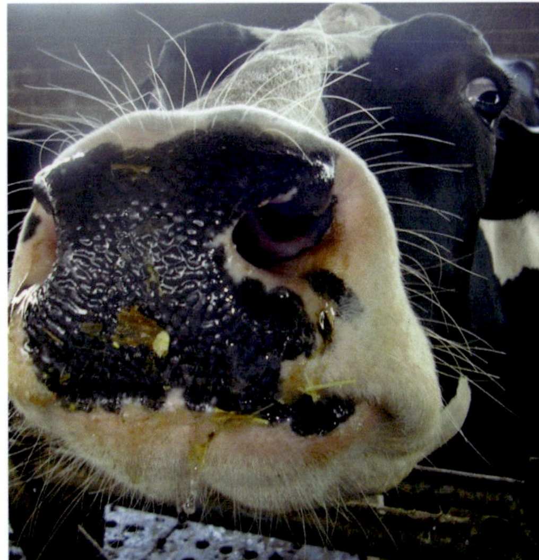

Hypothalamic-pituitary-gonadal axis

Hormones act as chemical mediators that trigger a cascade of events: the hypothalamus synthesises releasing hormones (RH), which in turn target the pituitary. These hormones enter the bloodstream and, instead of passing into general circulation, are transported via the hypophyseal portal system (via capillaries).

Table 1. Releasing hormones.

GH-RH	Growth hormone (GH)-releasing hormone
LH-RH	In cattle these two hormones are considered jointly as GnRH (gonadotropin-releasing hormone)
FSH-RH	
Prolactin-RH	Prolactin-releasing hormone (PRL)
CRH	Adrenocorticotropic hormone (ACTH)
TRH	Thyrotropin-releasing hormone (TSH)

Table 2. Hormones released from the pituitary upon the arrival of releasing hormones.

Anterior lobe	Posterior lobe
• Gonadotropic hormones (FSH-LH). • Prolactin (PRL). • Growth hormone (GH). • Adrenocorticotropic hormone (ACTH). • Thyrotropic hormone (TSH).	• Oxytocin. • Vasopressin (ADH).

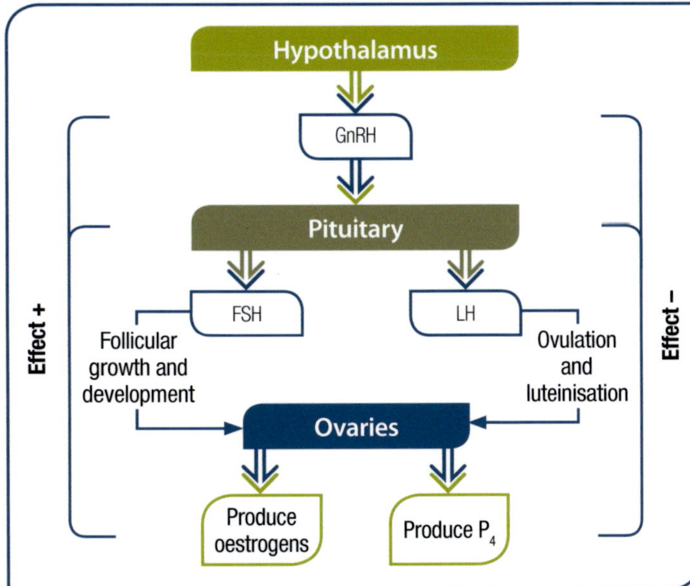

Figure 12. Feedback mechanisms that regulate the release of hormones in the hypothalamus-pituitary-gonadal axis.

The cycle ends with the release of the oocyte at ovulation

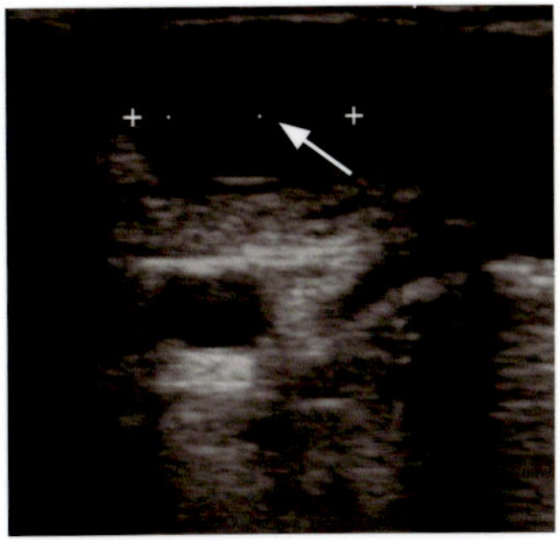

Figure 13. Measurement of dominant follicle (2.4 cm).

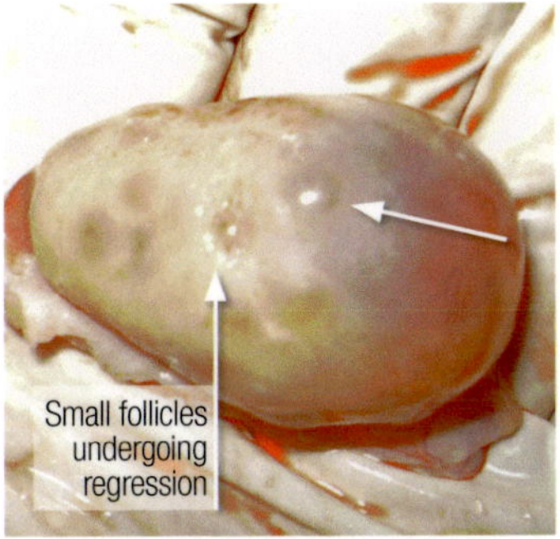

Figure 14. Preovulatory follicle (arrow).

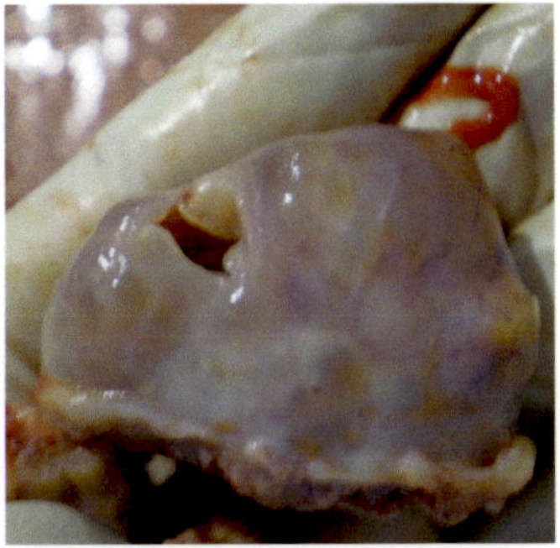

Figure 15. Thinning of the follicle wall and rupture of the stigma. This creates a gap through which the ovarian bursa passes by gravity, from where it is directed towards the horn by the movement of ciliated cells.

Follicular waves

- The follicular population in the ovary follows a dynamic that reflects the growth and regression of follicles on their path towards the formation of the preovulatory follicle.
- The oestrous cycle of the cow (18-24 days) is characterised by 1 to 4 waves of follicular growth (most commonly 2 and sometimes 3 waves, and even 4 waves).

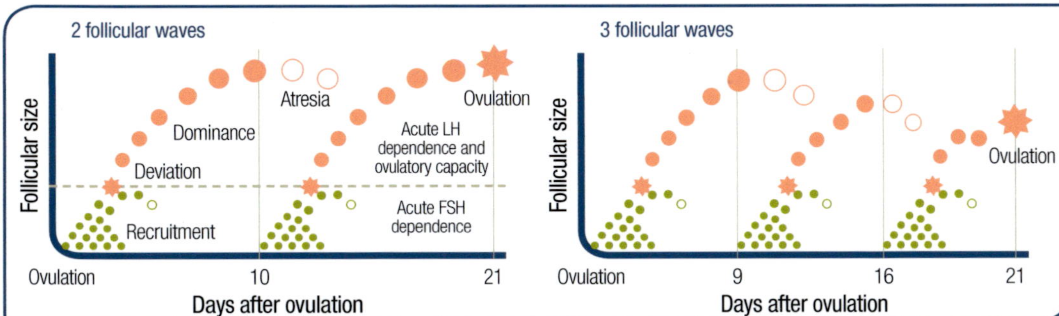

Figure 16. 2 and 3 follicular waves, respectively (Fricke, 2010).

Changes in the physiology of the new corpus luteum parallel the waves of follicular growth

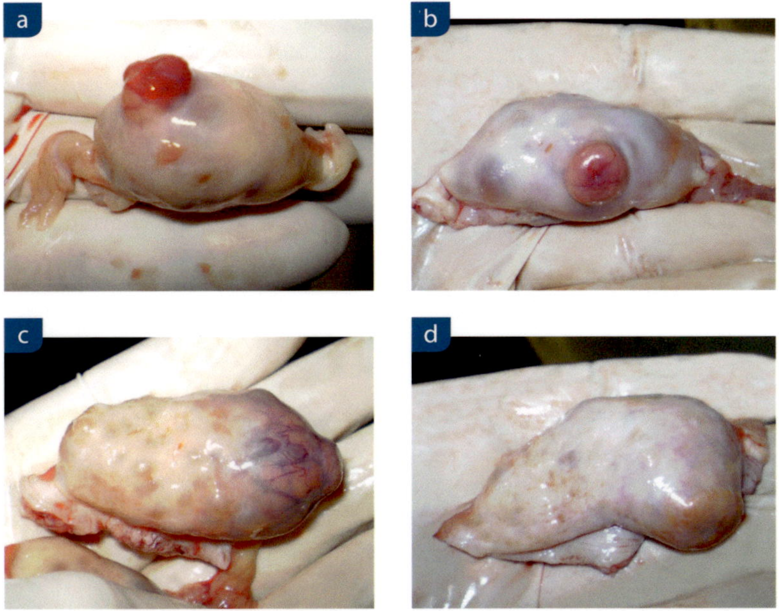

Figure 17. Corpora lutea at different stages of growth: (a and b) young corpus luteum (deep red color); (c) a full-sized, highly-irrigated corpus luteum; and (d) a less smooth and paler corpus luteum.

Phases of each wave of follicular growth

- Two waves

Recruitment (days 2-3): growth of a group of gonadotropin-dependent follicles of at least 2 mm in diameter caused by a transient increase in FSH.

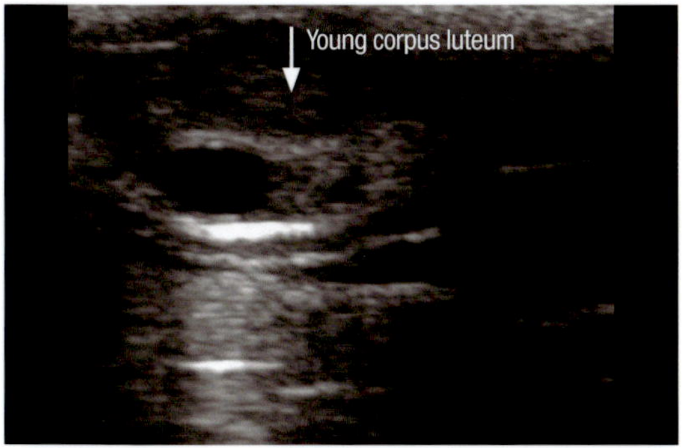

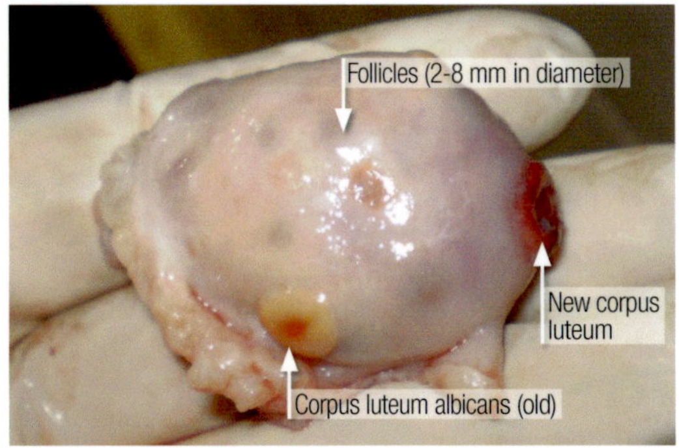

Figure 18. Recruitment of follicles of 2-8 mm in diameter.

First wave

Selection (days 3-5): one or more follicles emerge from among those recruited.

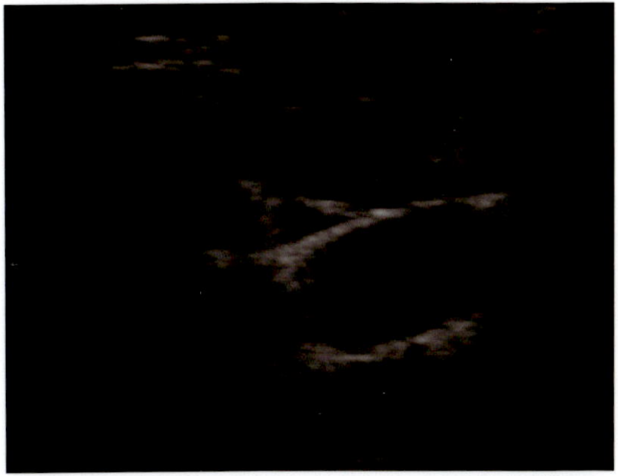

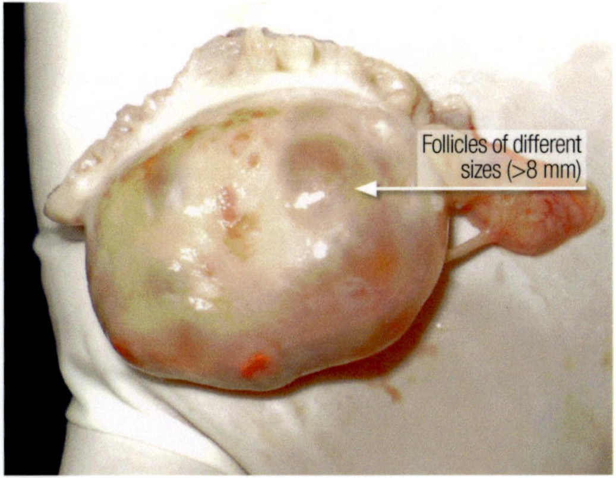

Figure 19. The concentration of circulating FSH is lower than that which induced recruitment, resulting in atresia of the recruited follicles, except for the selected follicle, which persists, via different mechanisms, despite the decrease in FSH (deviation).

Dominance (days 6-10): follicular dominance is both morphological (exerted by the largest follicle) and functional.

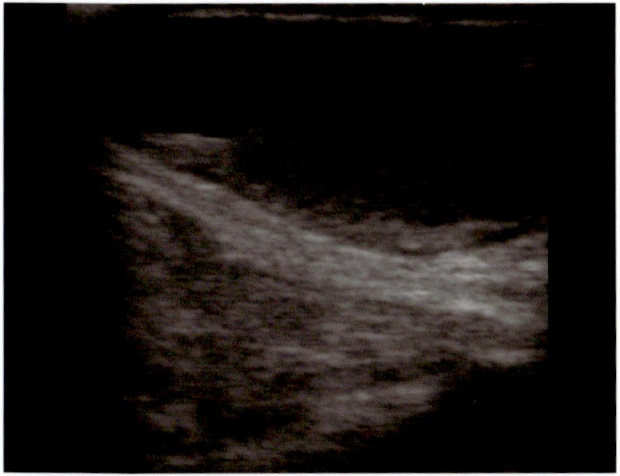

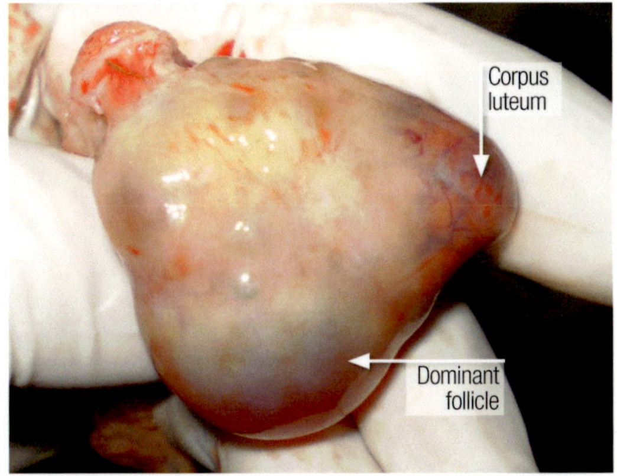

Figure 20. The follicle will not ovulate in the presence of P_4 secreted by the corpus luteum, and will undergo atresia and eventually disappear.

Dominance (days 11-12): dominant corpus luteum and small follicles, possibly undergoing recruitment.

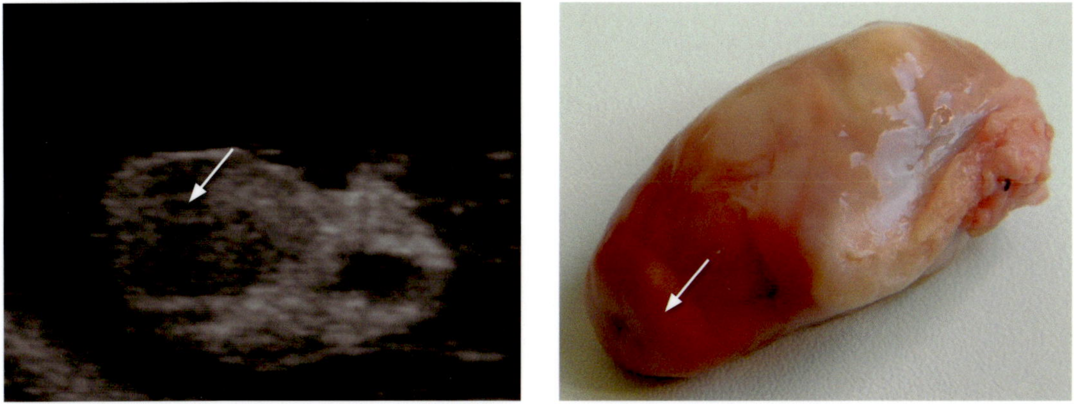

Figure 21. This phase is difficult to distinguish from the previous phase. It is more common to observe several follicular structures of varying sizes than small follicles potentially undergoing recruitment.

- Second wave

Recruitment/selection (days 13-18): follicular dominance is both morphological (exerted by the largest follicle) and functional.

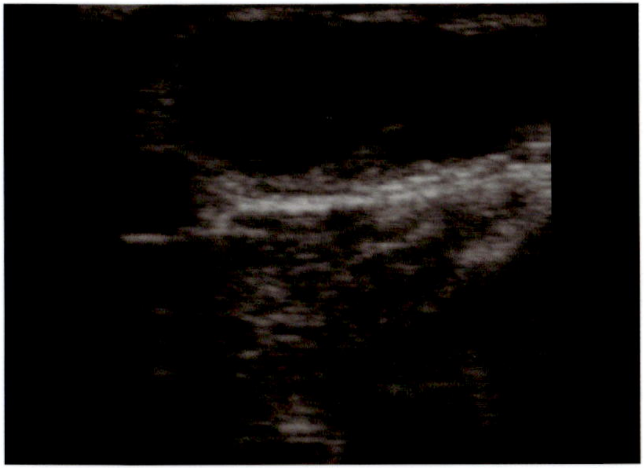

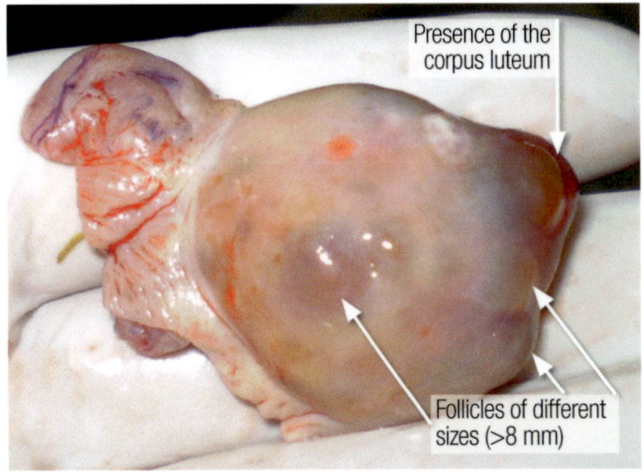

Figure 22. It is difficult to distinguish recruitment from selection during the second wave as the dominant follicle from the first wave, which has returned to its original size, persists.

Dominance (days 19-21): the dominant follicle reaches 20-25 mm, inducing oestrus and ovulation.

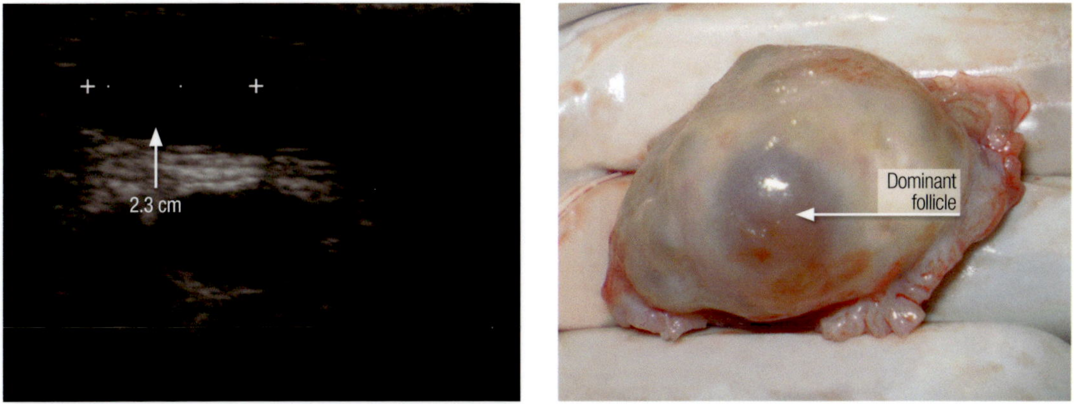

Figure 23. The cycle ends with the release of the oocyte at ovulation after the surge of LH.

Assessment and diagnosis of reproductive status

- The two ovaries are interdependent and function as if they were a single organ. Therefore, when studying structures, both ovaries should be evaluated, as evaluation of only a single ovary will result in an incomplete diagnosis.
- Parallel to the waves of follicular growth, the new corpus luteum, produced from the most recent ovulation, can be observed, as well as scar tissue and the remains (corpus albicans) of previous corpora lutea.
- Ultrasonography of the uterine horns provides sufficient information to resolve any doubts that may arise.

Methodology

Assessment

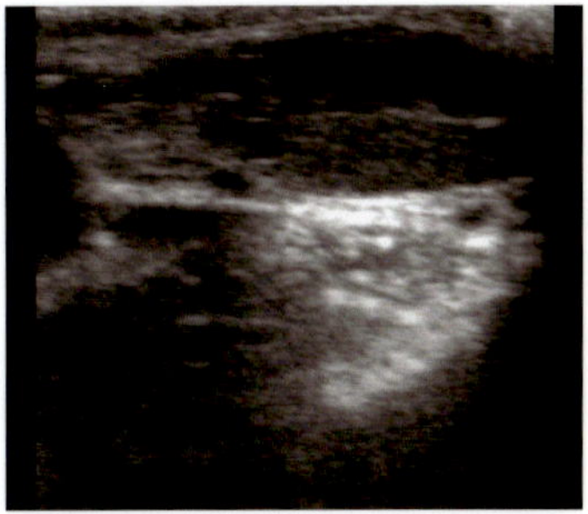

Figure 24. Right ovary: corpus luteum occupying almost the entire ovary.

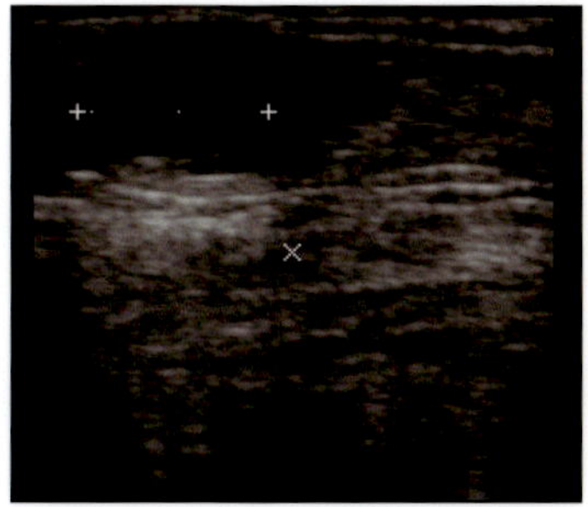

Figure 25. Left ovary: dominant follicle.

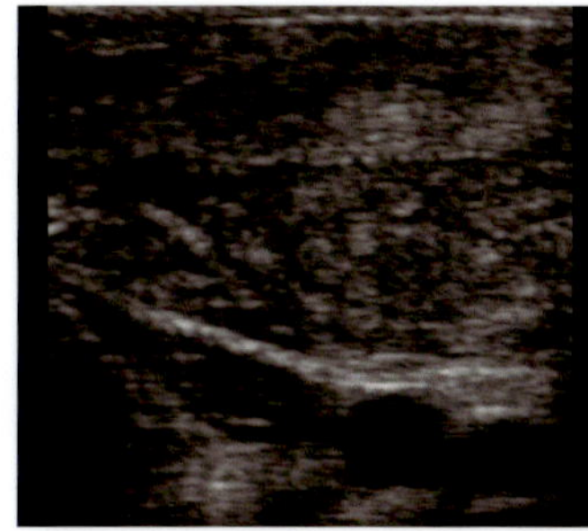

Figure 26. Uterine horns: endometrium and myometrium are of comparable sizes.

Evaluation

Cow in dominant phase of the first wave: ovulation will not occur due to the levels of P_4 generated by the corpus luteum.

Assessment of the uterus

Before and after heat (pro-oestrus and metoestrus), the endometrium (red arrows) occupies more space than the myometrium (white arrows), while mid-cycle (dioestrus) both occupy a similar amount of space.

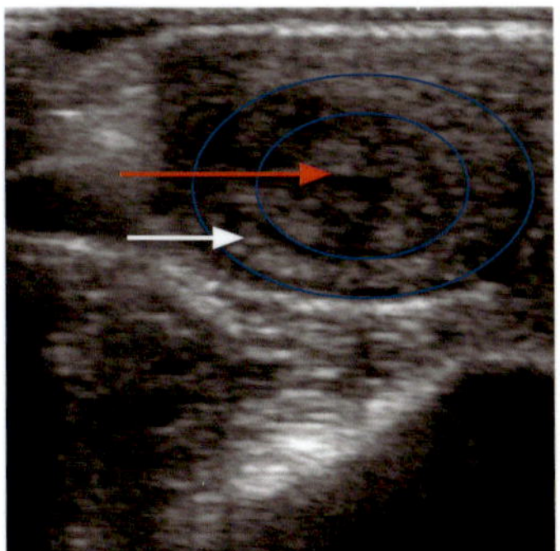

Figure 27. Metoestrus (days 1-5).

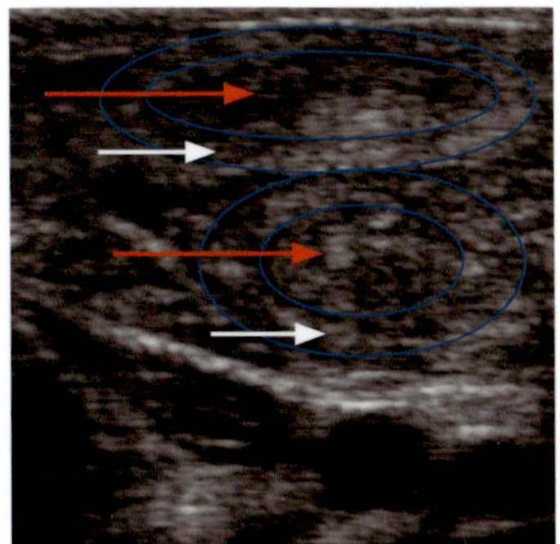

Figure 28. Dioestrus (days 6-17).

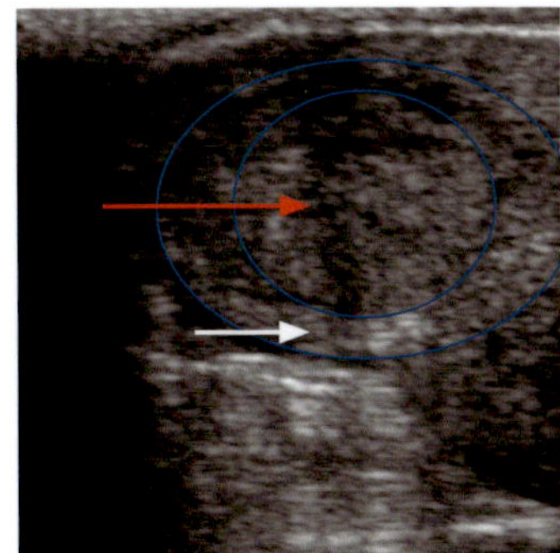

Figure 29. Pro-oestrus (days 18-21).

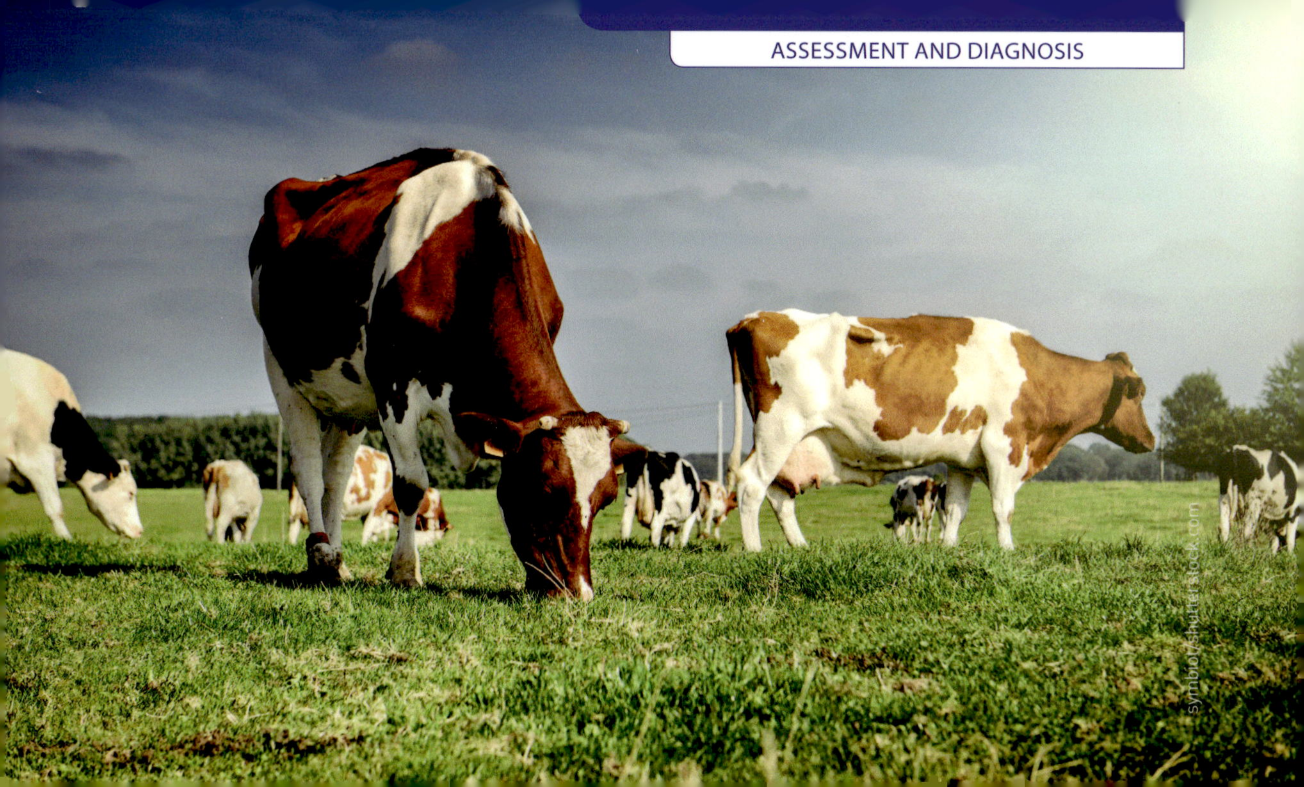

symbiot/shutterstock.com

Case studies

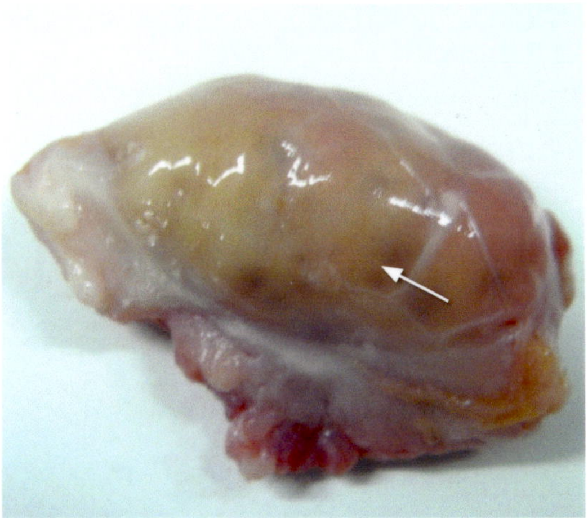

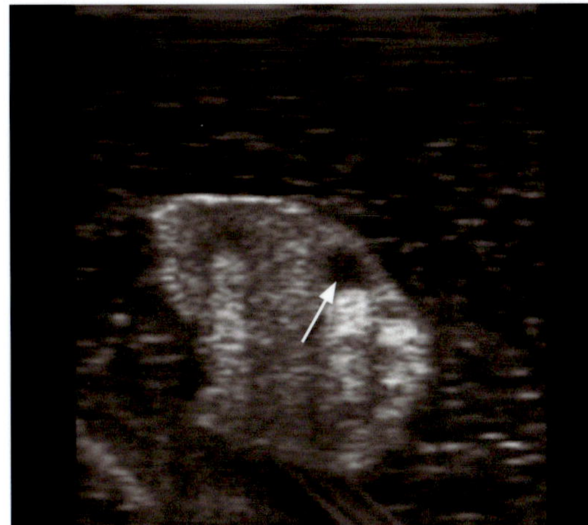

Figure 30. Recruitment of follicles (arrows) (2-5 days).

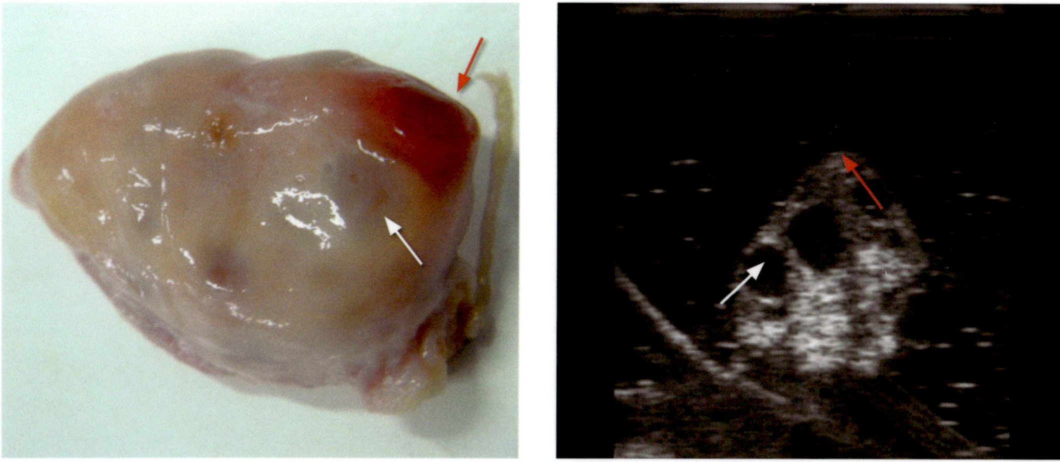

Figure 31. Young corpus luteum (red arrows) and follicles in selection phase (white arrows) (2-5 days).

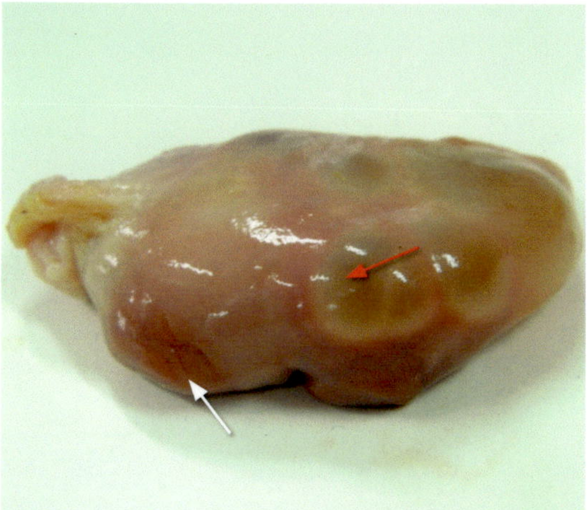

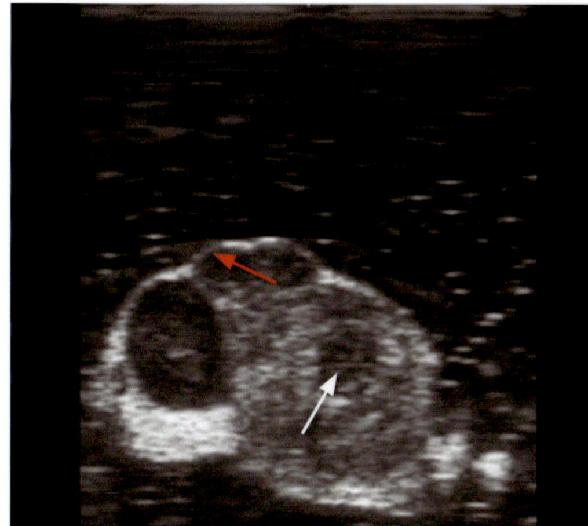

Figure 32. Follicles in selection phase (red arrows) and corpus luteum with cavity (white arrows) (6-10 days).

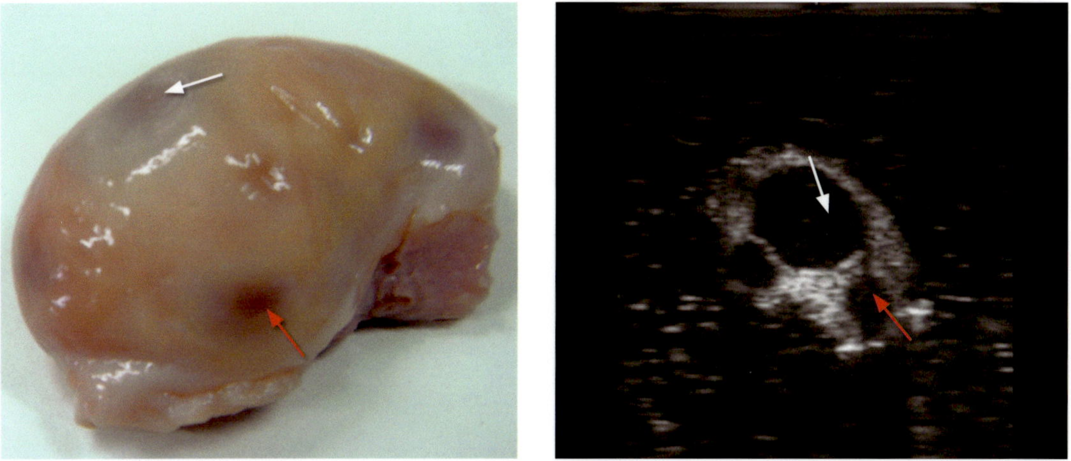

Figure 33. Follicles in selection phase (red arrows) (note prominent follicle [white arrows]) (6-10 days).

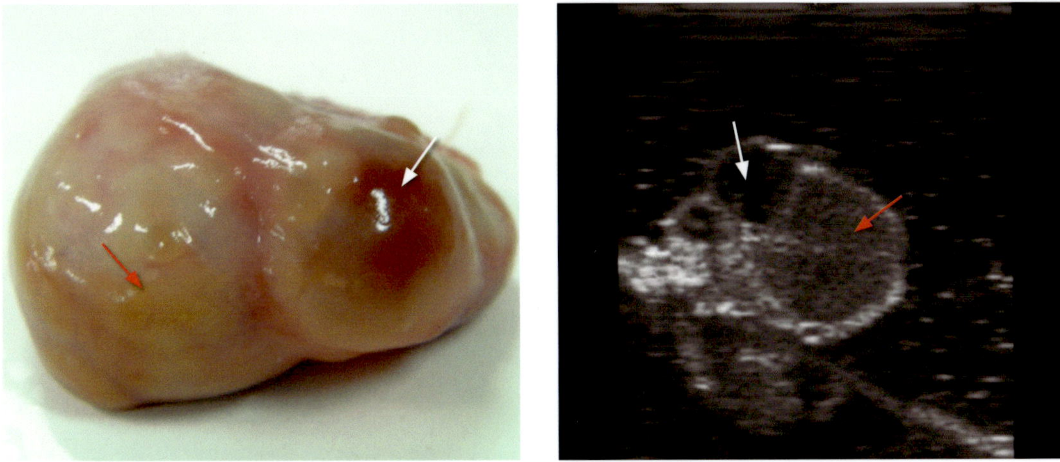

Figure 34. Corpus luteum (red arrows) and prominent follicle (white arrows) (6-10 days).

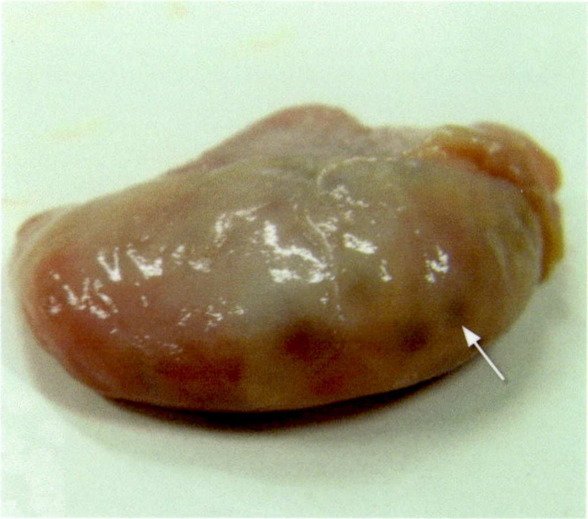

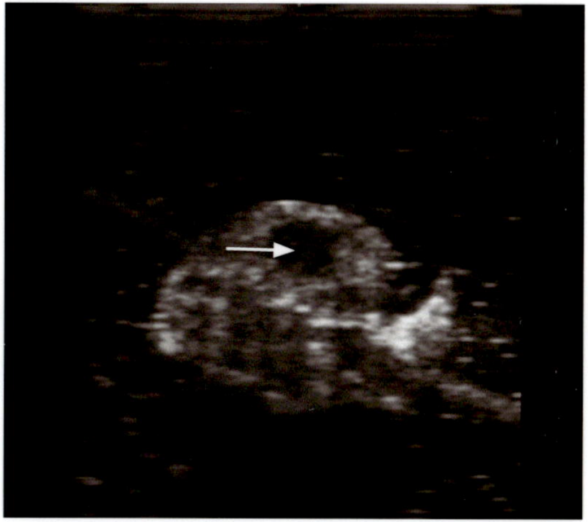

Figure 35. Follicles of various sizes (arrows) (6-10 days).

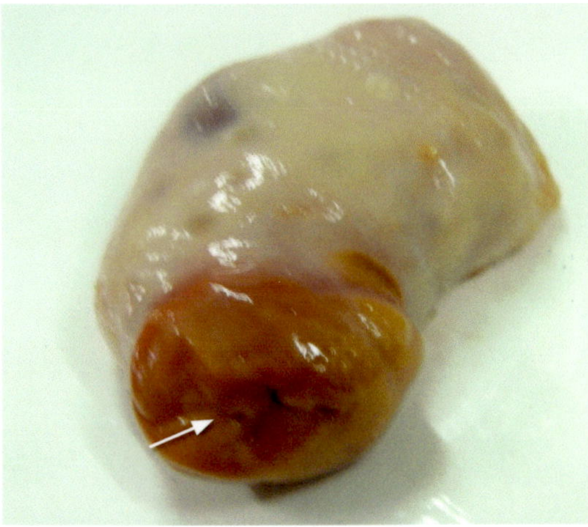

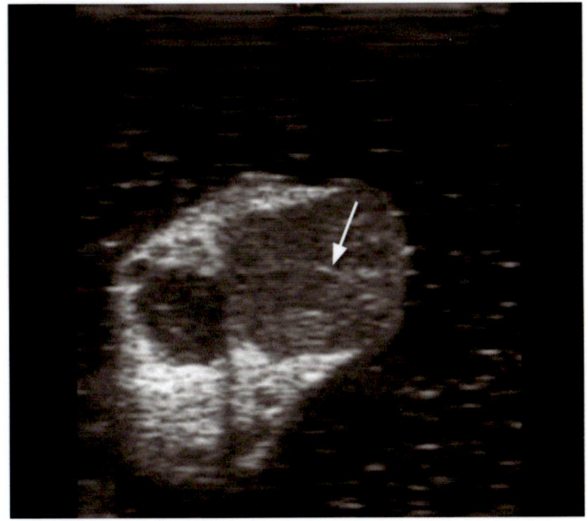

Figure 36. Prominent corpus luteum (arrows) (11-12 days).

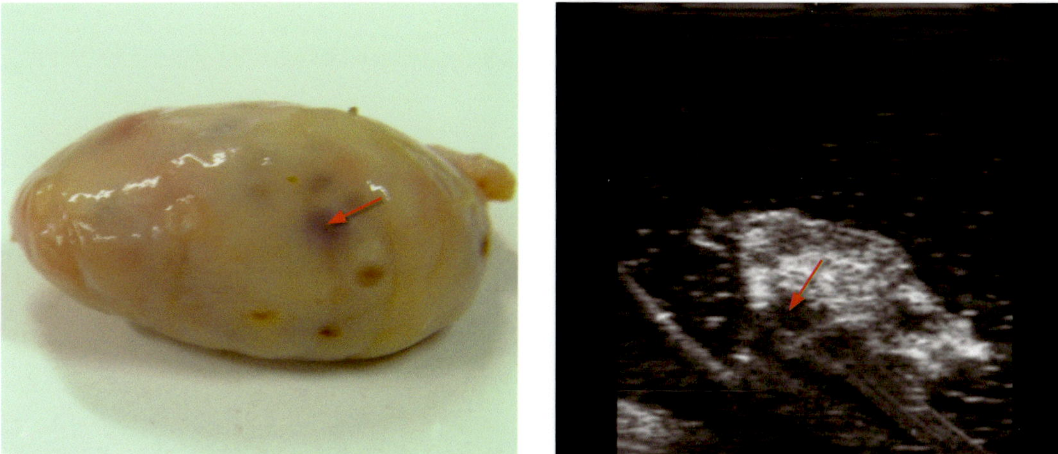

Figure 37. Follicles in recruitment/selection phase (arrows) (11-12 days).

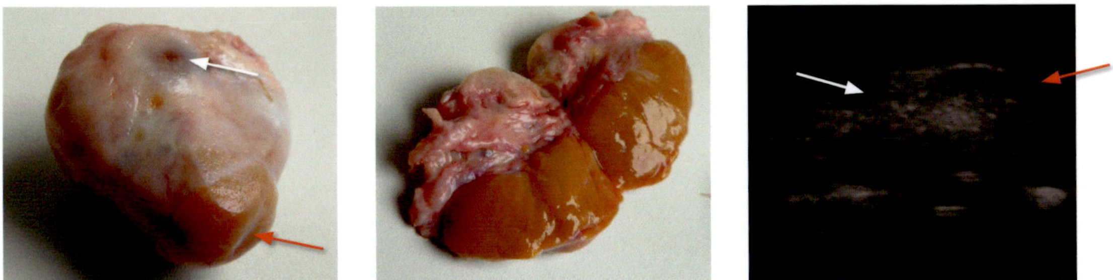

Figure 38. Corpus luteum (red arrows) and follicle (not very prominent, white arrows) (11-12 days).

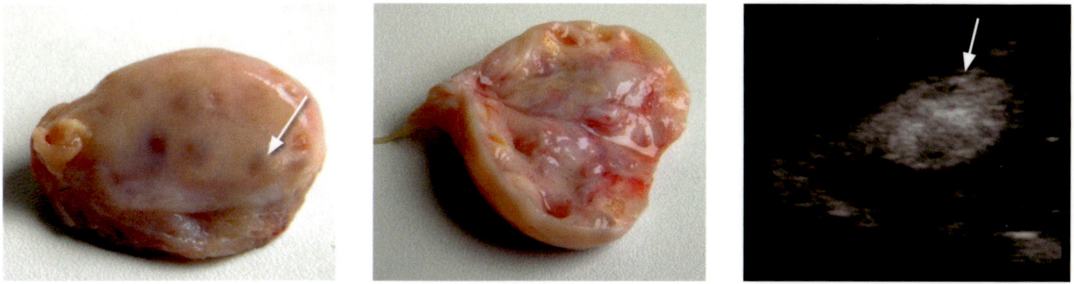

Figure 39. Small follicles (arrows) (11-12 days).

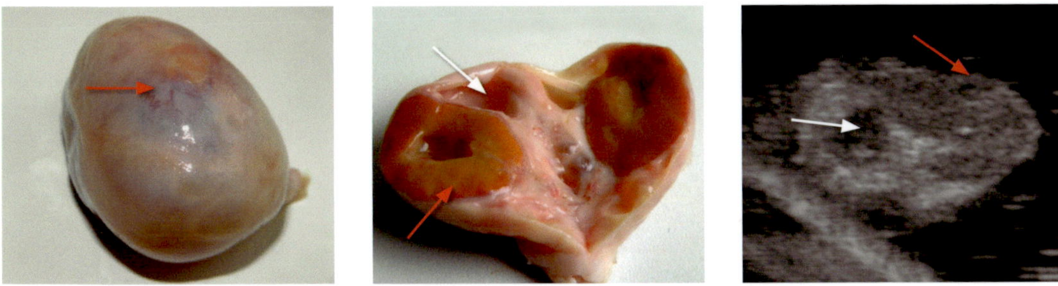

Figure 40. Corpus luteum with prominent cavity (red arrows) and follicle (white arrows) (6-10 days).

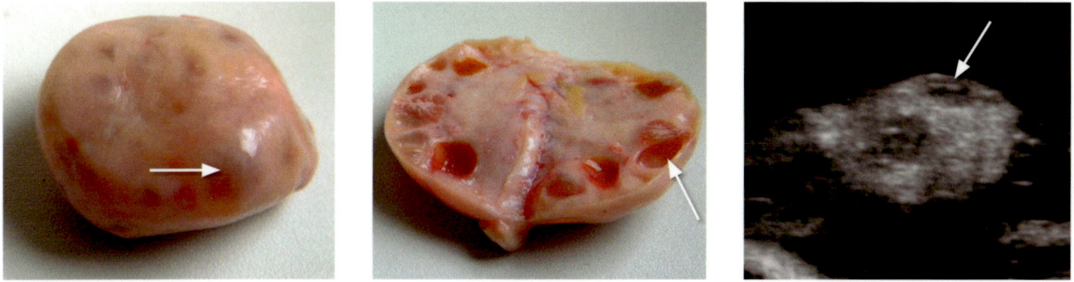

Figure 41. Small follicles (arrows) (6-10 days).

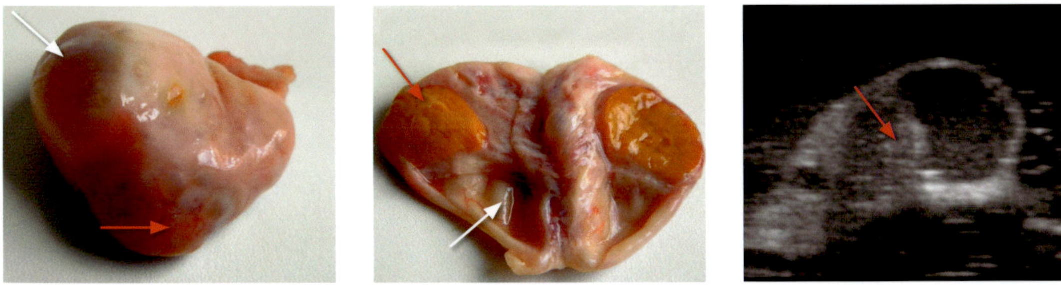

Figure 42. Prominent corpus luteum (red arrows) and follicle (white arrows) (6-10 days).

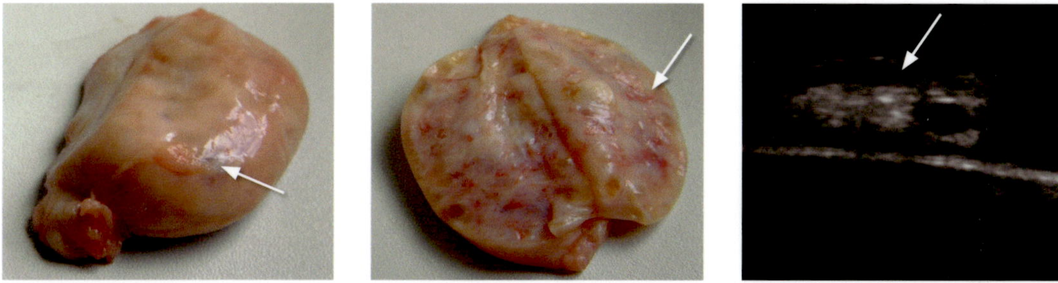

Figure 43. Small follicles (arrows) (6-10 days).

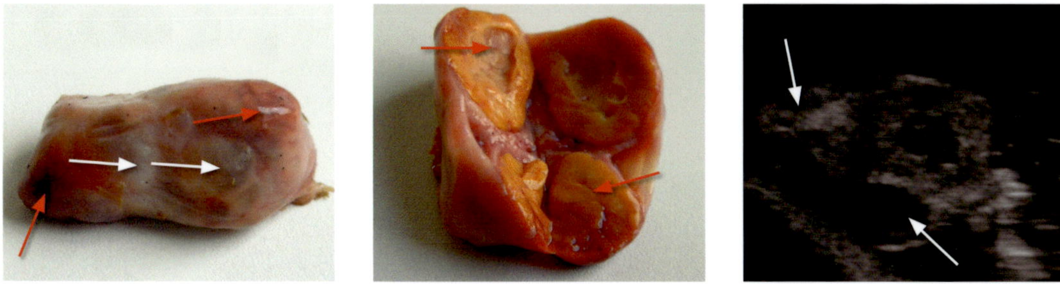

Figure 44. Two corpora lutea (red arrows), one of which contains a cavity (double ovulation occurred in the previous cycle), and follicles of varying sizes (white arrows) (11-12 days).

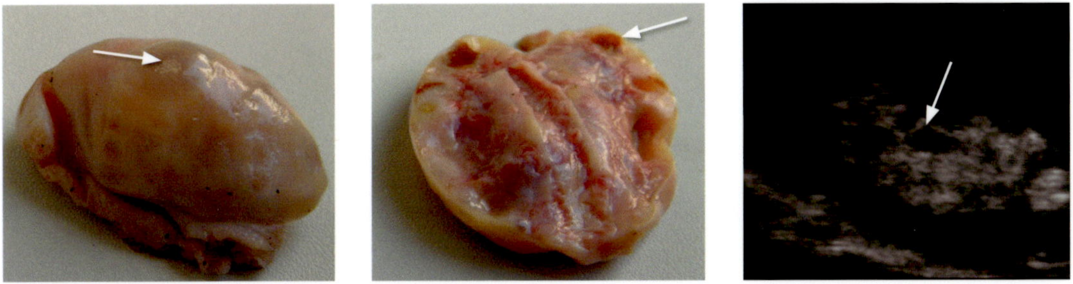

Figure 45. Small follicles clustered in the cortex (arrows) (11-12 days).

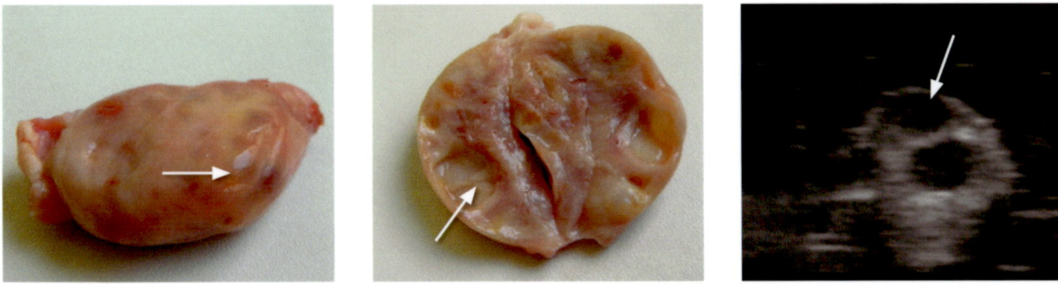

Figure 46. Follicles of varying sizes (arrows) (2-3 days).

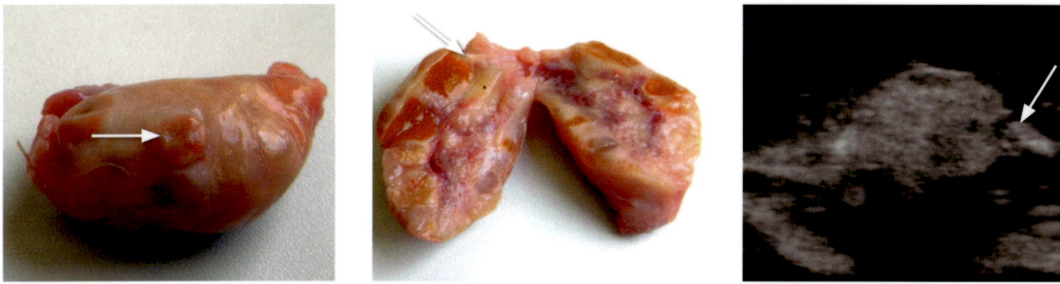

Figure 47. Scars of old corpora lutea (arrows) and low-level follicular activity (2-3 days).

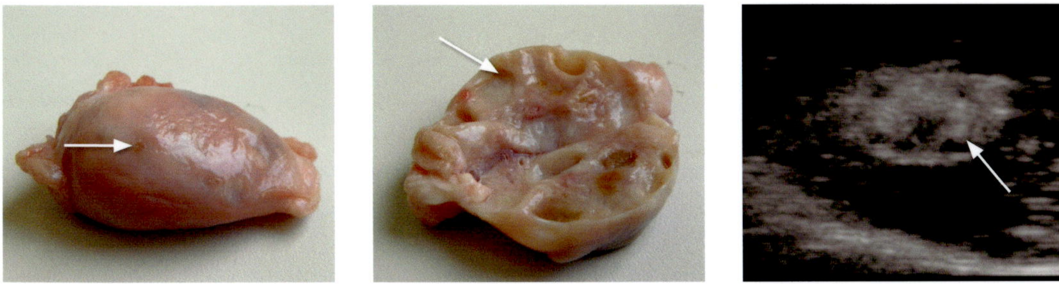

Figure 48. Follicles of varying sizes (arrows) (19-21 days).

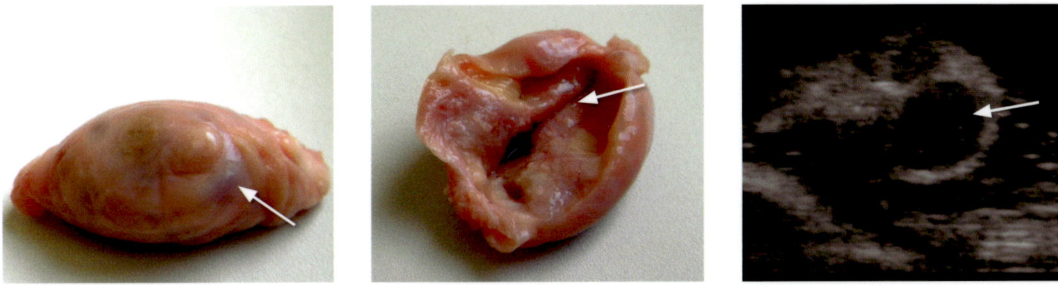

Figure 49. Dominant follicle (arrows) (19-21 days).

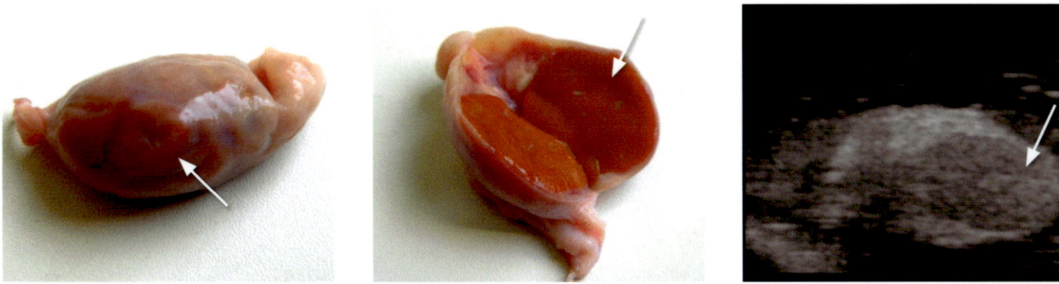

Figure 50. Prominent corpus luteum (arrows) (13-18 days).

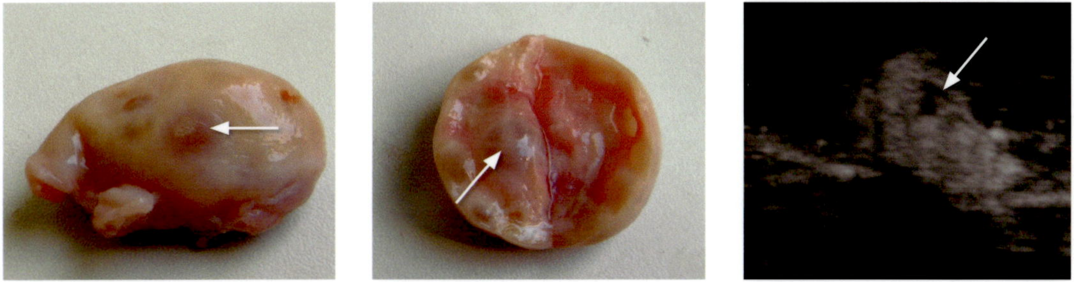

Figure 51. Follicles of varying sizes (arrows) (13-18 days).

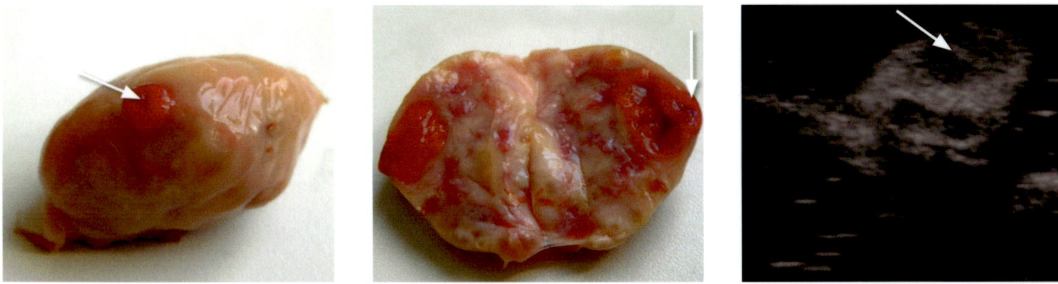

Figure 52. Young corpus luteum beginning development (arrows) (2-3 days).

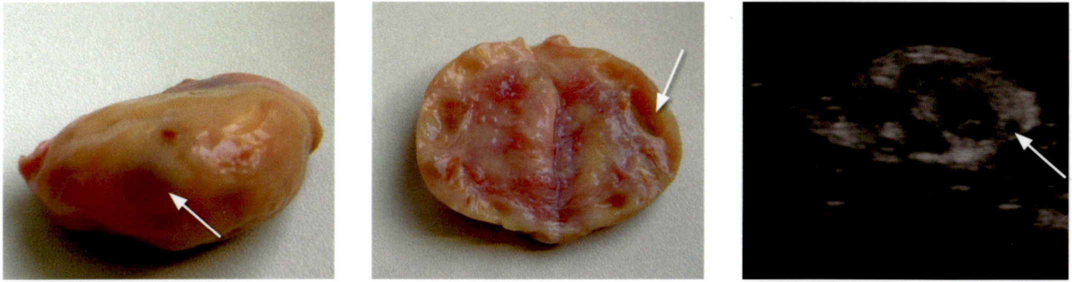

Figure 53. Follicles of varying sizes (arrows) (2-3 days).

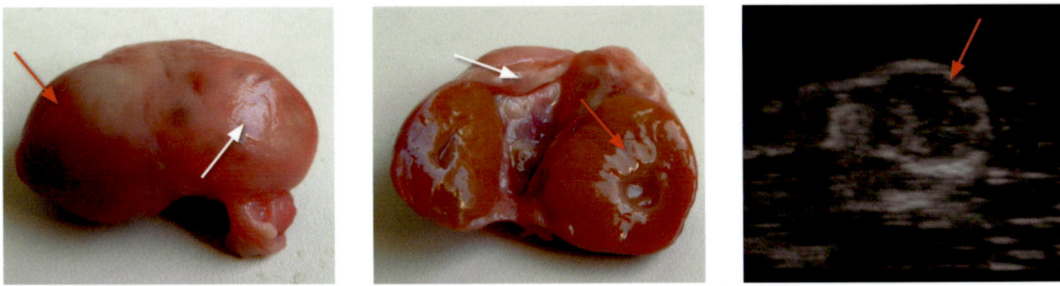

Figure 54. Prominent follicle (white arrows) and corpus luteum with cavity (red arrows) (6-10 days).

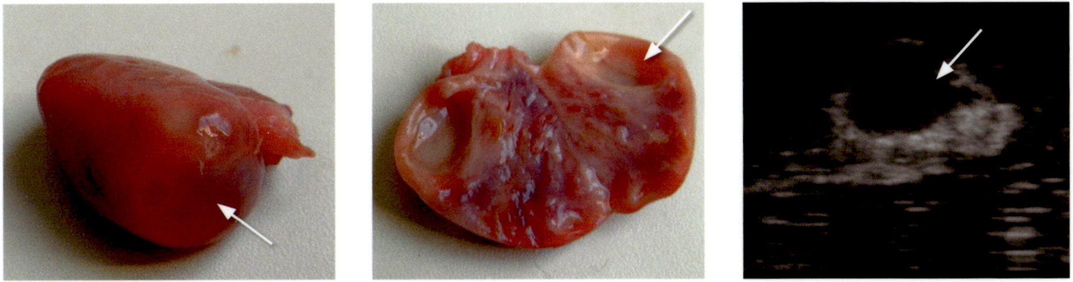

Figure 55. Dominant follicle (arrows) (6-10 days).

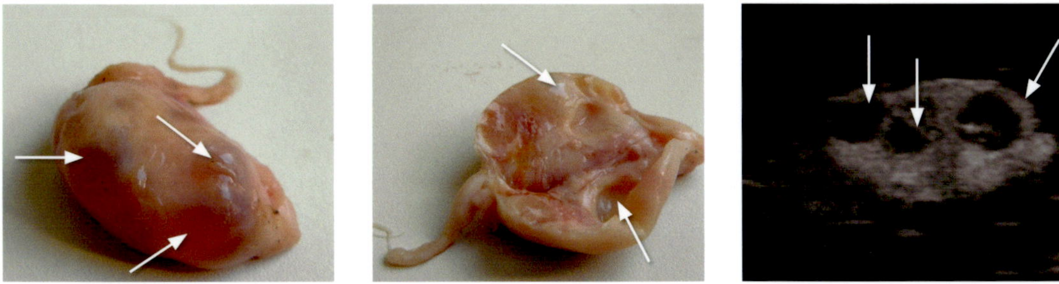

Figure 56. Follicles of varying sizes (arrows) (2-3 days).

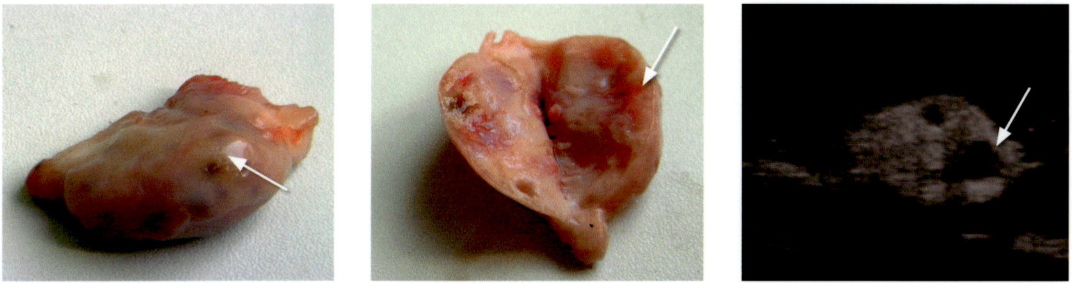

Figure 57. Small follicles (arrows) (2-3 days).

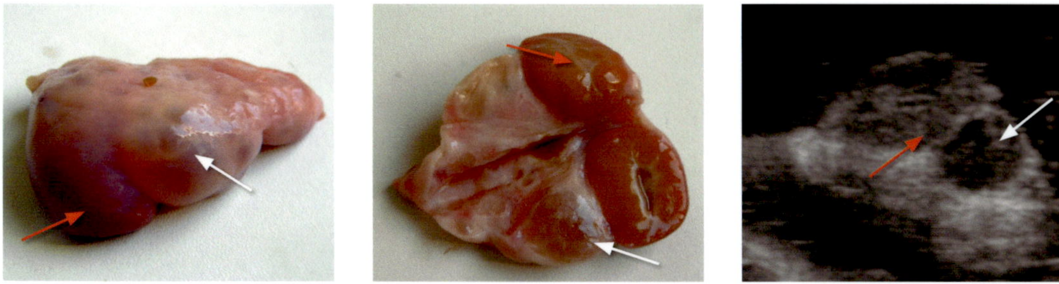

Figure 58. Prominent corpus luteum (red arrows) and dominant follicle (white arrows) (6-10 days).

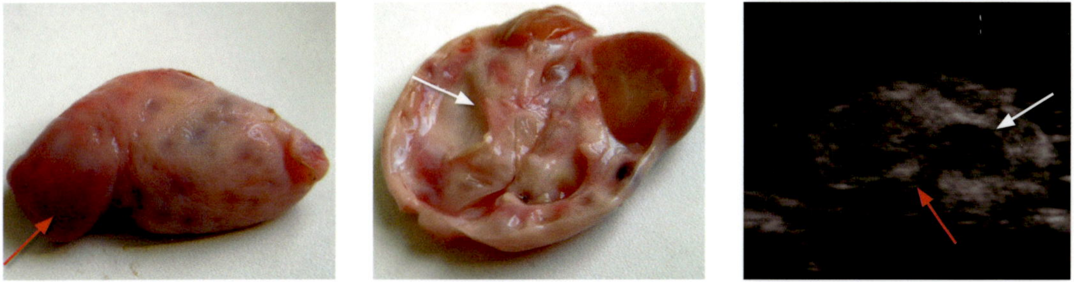

Figure 59. Prominent corpus luteum (red arrows) and several follicles, one of which is prominent (white arrows) (6-10 days).

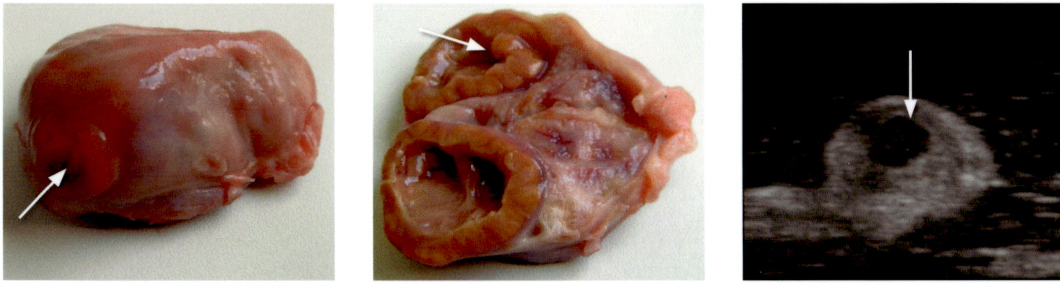

Figure 60. Corpus luteum with cavity (arrows) (3-5 days).

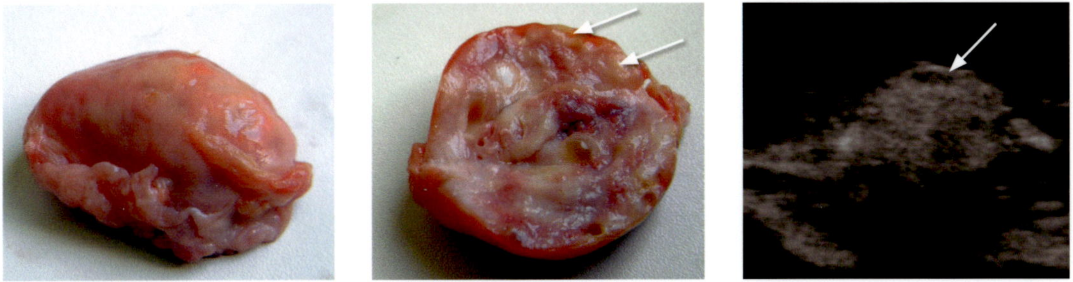

Figure 61. Small follicles (arrows) (3-5 days).

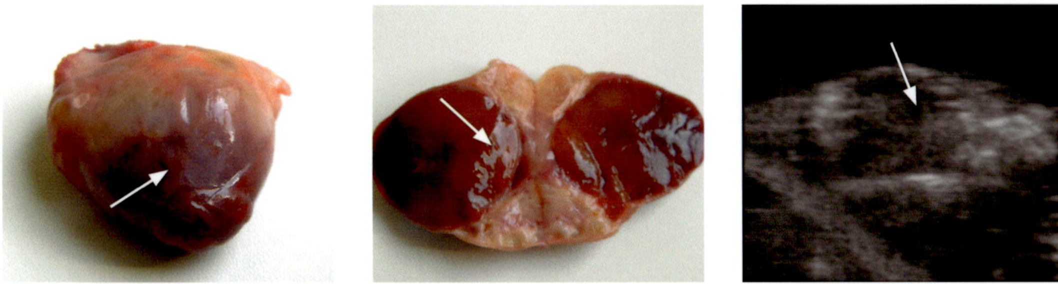

Figure 62. Very prominent corpus luteum (arrows) (6-10 days).

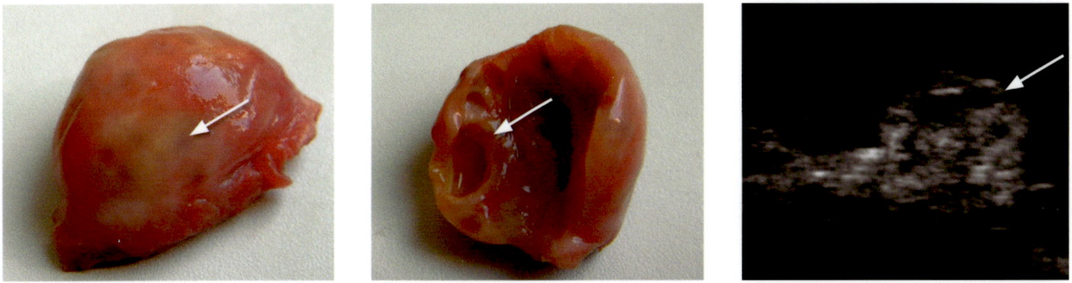

Figure 63. Several follicles of varying sizes (arrows) (6-10 days).

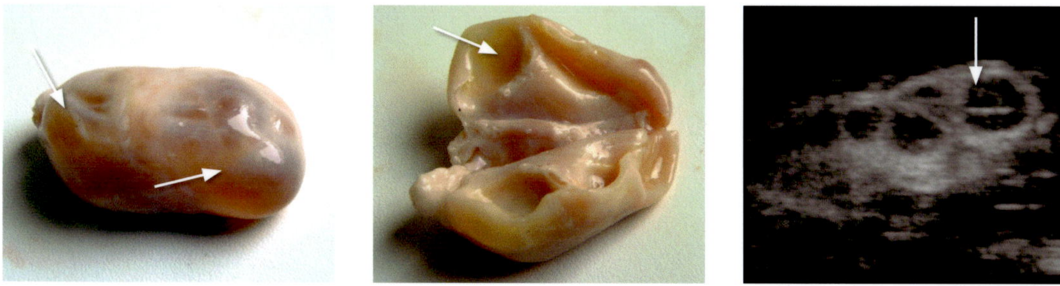

Figure 64. Several prominent follicles of about 2 cm (arrows) (19-21 days).

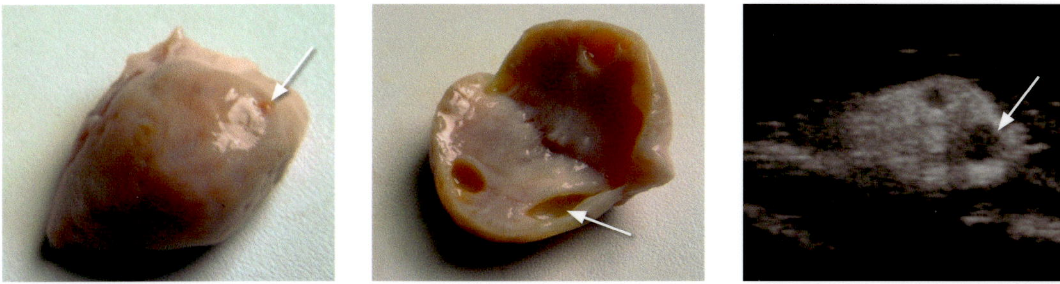

Figure 65. Small follicles clustered in the cortex (arrows) (19-21 days).

Follicular cyst

- Persists >10 days.
- Diameter >10 mm.
- Monolateral or bilateral.
- Similar to follicle but larger.
- Normally, there is no corpus luteum (it may appear in up to 30 % of cases: without endocrine activity).

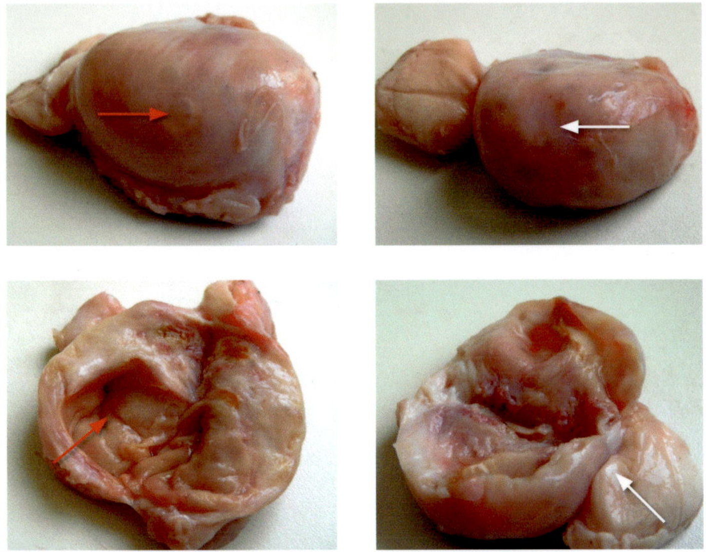

Figure 66. Follicular cyst (red arrows) and prominent follicle (white arrows).

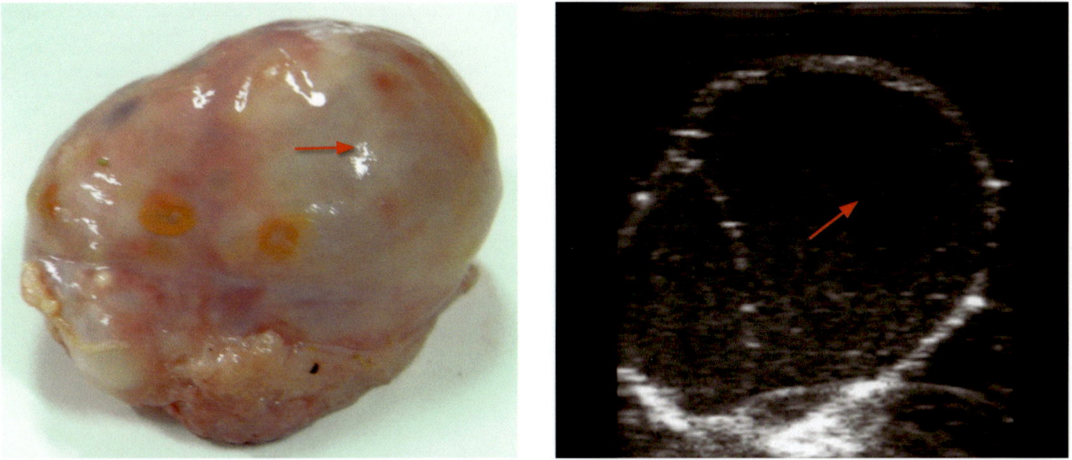

Figure 67. Follicular cyst (with two cavities) (6 cm) (arrows).

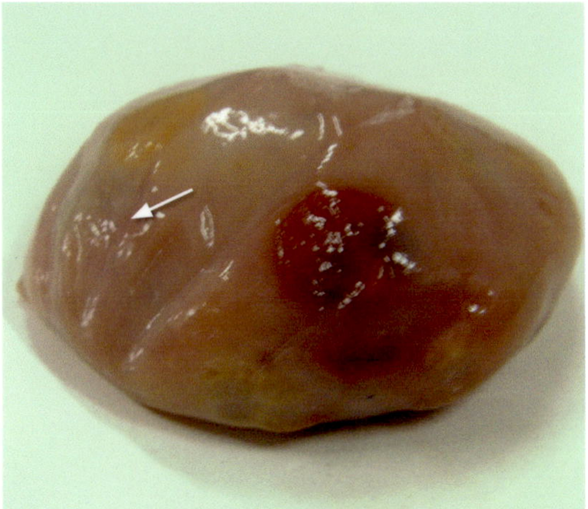

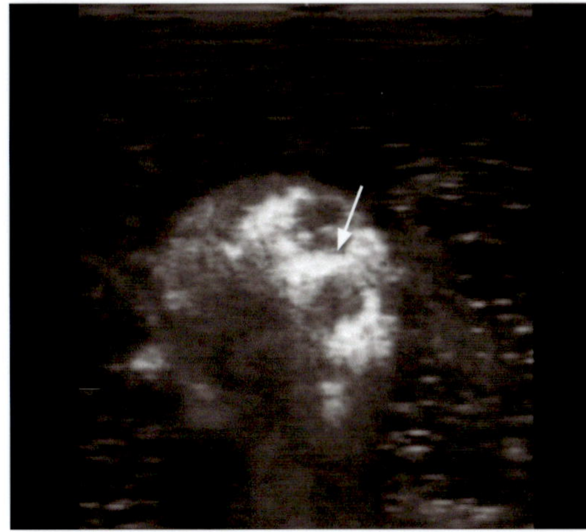

Figure 68. Follicles (arrows).

Luteal cyst

- Wall of 1-3 mm.
- Persists >10 days.
- Cavity of >10 mm in diameter.
- Monolateral.

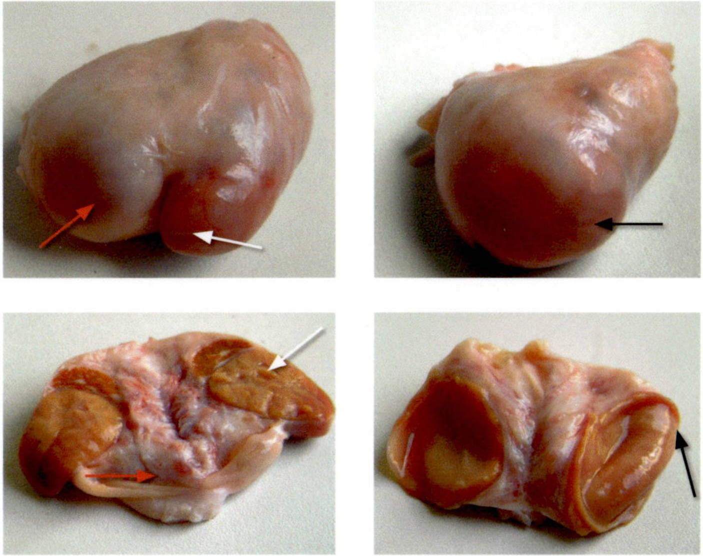

Figure 69. Prominent follicle in the left ovary (red arrows) accompanied by a prominent corpus luteum (white arrows), and a luteal cyst in the right ovary (wall thickness >3 mm) (black arrows).

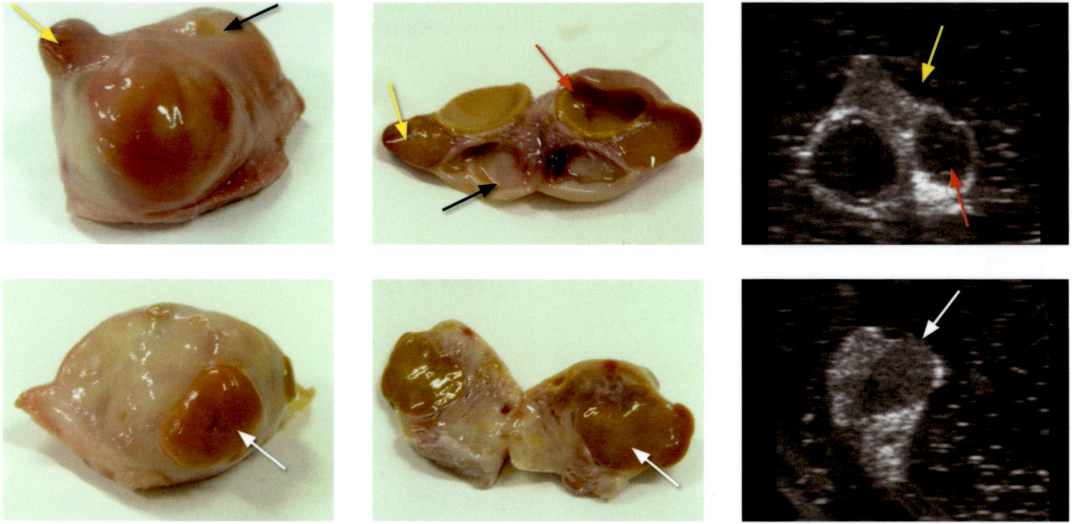

Figure 70. Wall of luteal cyst (red arrows), corpus luteum (yellow arrows), and prominent follicle (black arrows) in left ovary. Corpus luteum (white arrows) in right ovary.